The

Inspired Alkaline

Diet

Easy Alkaline Recipes to Boost your Diet

Sam Carter

I0145984

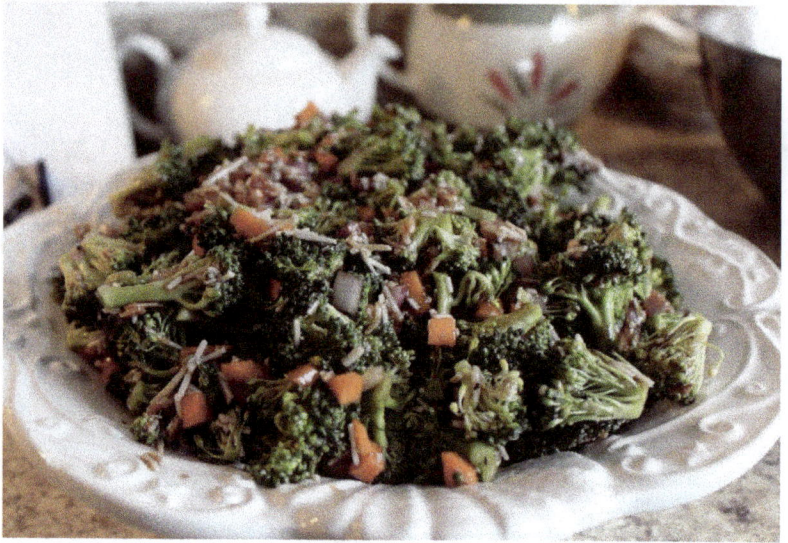

© **Copyright 2021 - All rights reserved.**

The content contained within this book may not be reproduced, duplicated or transmitted without direct written permission from the author or the publisher.

Under no circumstances will any blame or legal responsibility be held against the publisher, or author, for any damages, reparation, or monetary loss due to the information contained within this book. Either directly or indirectly.

Legal Notice:

This book is copyright protected. This book is only for personal use. You cannot amend, distribute, sell, use, quote or paraphrase any part, or the content within this book, without the consent of the author or publisher.

Disclaimer Notice:

Please note the information contained within this document is for educational and entertainment purposes only. All effort has been executed to present accurate, up to date, and reliable, complete information. No warranties of any kind are declared or implied. Readers acknowledge that the author is not engaging in the rendering of legal, financial, medical or professional advice. The content within this book has been derived from various sources. Please consult a licensed professional before attempting any techniques outlined in this book.

By reading this document, the reader agrees that under no circumstances is the author responsible for any losses, direct or indirect, which are incurred as a result of the use of information contained within this document, including, but not limited to, — errors, omissions, or inaccuracies.

Table of Contents

Meatless Taco Wraps 7

Quinoa & Black Sesame Pilaf 9

Sweet Potato Stew 13

Cashew Zoodles 15

Butternut Squash Risotto 17

Meatless Meatloaf Cups 19

Spicy Dal & Greens 22

Blackened Salmon with Fruit Salsa 24

Roasted Cauliflower with Chimichurri Sauce 26

Cook-off Chili 29

Pasta & Veggie Stroganoff 31

Tofu Mole with Jicama Salad 33

Tricolor Pasta 38

Cauliflower Pasta Pillows in Red Sauce 40

Raw Thai Curry 43

Shrimp & Arugula Salad 45

Avocado and Tomato Pizza 47

Spinach Ravioli 49

Kale & Squash Vegetable Gratin 52

Spicy Orange Sweet Potato Bowl 55

Cauliflower Colcannon 57

Peas & Rice 59

Sweet & Spicy Sweet Potato Skillet 61

Broccoli & Pear Salad 63

Quinoa Niçoise Salad 65

Red & Green Salad 67

Shredded Kale Salad 69

Italian Kale Stew 71

Spinach & Beet Salad 73

Spicy Cabbage Bowl 75

Fennel Citrus Salad 77

Salmon & Vegetable Kebabs with Greens Pesto 79

Coconut Curry & Vegetables 81

Loaded Spaghetti Squash 83

Asian Noodle Bowl 85

Spicy Marinara Sauce & Pasta 87

Lemon Baked Fish Over Green Salad 89

Cauliflower & Tahini Bowl 91

Stuffed Peppers 93

Raw Beetroot Lasagna 95

Baba Ganoush Pasta 97

"Cheesy" Broccoli Bowl 99

Lentil & Green Bean Pesto Salad 100

Vegetable Packed Minestrone 102

Noodle Soup with Greens 104

Southwest Tofu Burger 106

Zucchini Rolls with Red Sauce 108

Meatless Taco Wraps

Servings: 2

Total Time: 20 minutes

Ingredients

- 1 ½ cups brown lentils, cooked

- ½ cup walnuts, toasted

- 1 tablespoon tomato paste

- 1 garlic clove, minced

- ½ teaspoon smoked paprika

- ½ teaspoon chili powder

- ½ teaspoon cumin

- ½ teaspoon Himalayan salt

- ¼ cup water

- 4 romaine leaves

- ½ avocado, sliced

Rainbow Salsa

- ½ cup mango, diced

- ½ cup red bell pepper, diced

- ½ cup green bell pepper, diced

- 3 tablespoons cilantro, chopped

- 1 tablespoon apple cider vinegar

- ½ teaspoon Himalayan salt

- ½ teaspoon black pepper, crushed

Directions

1. Make Rainbow Salsa by placing all Rainbow Salsa ingredients in a medium bowl and stirring to combine. Let sit for 10 minutes while you make the taco meat.

2. In a food processor, pulse together the lentils, walnuts, tomato paste, garlic, paprika, chili powder, cumin, salt and water. The mixture should be crumbly and not overly smooth.

3. Place the lentil & walnut mixture into each of the romaine leaves and top with Rainbow Salsa and avocado slices.

Quinoa & Black Sesame Pilaf

Servings: 2

Total Time: 25 minutes

Ingredients

- 1 cup green beans, trimmed and cut into 1 inch pieces
- 2 carrots, peeled and sliced into matchsticks
- 2 tablespoons olive oil, divided
- 2 teaspoons Himalayan salt, divided
- 2 teaspoons black pepper, crushed and divided
- 1 shallot, sliced
- 1 celery stalk, finely diced
- ½ cup green bell pepper, finely diced
- 1 garlic clove, minced
- ½ cup quinoa
- 1 cup vegetable broth or water
- 1 cup green lentils, cooked

Dressing

- 1/3 cup avocado oil
- 2 teaspoons toasted sesame oil

- 1 teaspoon fresh ginger, grated

- 1 teaspoon lemon zest

- ½ teaspoon red chili flakes

- ¼ cup tamari

- ¼ cup rice vinegar

- 2 tablespoons black sesame seeds, toasted

Directions

1. Place green beans and carrots on a parchment paper lined baking tray and drizzle with 1 tablespoon of olive oil, 1 teaspoon salt and 1 teaspoon black pepper. Cook under the broiler for about 5 minutes or until browned, turning about halfway through.

2. In a large pot, add remaining 1 tablespoon olive oil, shallot, celery, bell pepper and garlic, cooking for 5 minutes. Add quinoa, stirring to coat and cook 2 minutes, until toasted. Add broth or water, bring to a boil and then reduce heat and let simmer for 5 - 8 minutes or until liquid is absorbed.

3. To make dressing, add all dressing ingredients to a bowl and whisk to combine.

4. To assemble, mix together the lentils and quinoa. Season with remaining 1 teaspoon salt and 1 teaspoon pepper. Top with green bean and carrot mixture before drizzling dressing over entire dish.

Lemon Zucchini Pasta

Servings: 2

Total Time: 15 minutes

Ingredients

- 4 zucchinis
- 2 cups baby spinach, roughly chopped
- 1 cup kale, stems removed and roughly chopped
- ¼ cup fresh basil
- ¼ cup parsley
- 3 garlic cloves
- 1 lemon, juiced
- ¼ cup cashews, soaked overnight and drained
- 2 teaspoons red chili flakes
- 2 teaspoons lemon zest
- 1 cup olive oil
- 1 teaspoon Himalayan salt
- 1 teaspoon black pepper, crushed
- ½ cup cherry tomatoes, sliced in half
- ¼ cup pine nuts, toasted

Directions

1.   Using a spiralizer (or a vegetable peeler to make wider noodles), make zucchini into noodles and set aside.

2.   In a food processor combine the spinach, kale, basil, parsley, garlic, lemon juice, cashews, red chili flakes and lemon zest. Once finely chopped, slowly drizzle in olive oil.

3.   In a large bowl, toss together the zucchini noodles with the spinach/kale sauce. Season with salt and pepper before garnishing with tomatoes and pine nuts.

Sweet Potato Stew

Servings: 2

Total Time: 50 minutes

Ingredients

- 1 tablespoon olive oil

- ½ yellow onion, diced

- 2 garlic cloves, minced

- 1 tablespoon tomato paste

- 1 tablespoon apple cider vinegar

- ¼ cup rice flour

- 2 cups vegetable broth

- 1 tablespoon tamari

- 1 tablespoon coconut aminos

- 1 large carrot, cut into 1 inch pieces

- 1 cup sweet potatoes, cut into 1 inch chunks

- 1 stalk of celery, cut into ½ inch pieces

- 1 cup green peas, defrosted if frozen

- ½ tomato, diced

- 1 bay leaf

- 1 teaspoon black pepper

- 1 teaspoon dried thyme

- 1 teaspoon oregano

- ¼ cup parsley, chopped

Directions

1.   Heat oil in a large pot over medium heat. Add onion and garlic and cook for 5 minutes. Add tomato paste, vinegar and rice flour. Stir the mixture with a spoon consistently for 5 more minutes.

2.   Pour in broth, tamari and aminos and add carrot, sweet potato, celery, peas, tomato, bay leaf, pepper, thyme and oregano.

3.   Let come to a boil and then reduce heat to low and simmer for 20 minutes.

4.   After 10 minutes, stir in parsley and serve.

Cashew Zoodles

Servings: 2

Total Time: 30 minutes

Ingredients

- 1 small zucchini, cut into noodles with a spiralizer
- 1 yellow squash, cut into noodles with a spiralizer
- 1 ¼ teaspoon Himalayan salt
- 2 cups cashews, soaked overnight and drained
- 1 lemon, juiced
- 3 tablespoons water
- 2 tablespoons olive oil
- ¼ teaspoon turmeric
- 1 garlic clove
- 1 teaspoon onion powder
- 2 tablespoons nutritional yeast
- 1 teaspoon black pepper
- 10 cherry tomatoes, halved
- 2 teaspoons chives

Directions

1.   Place zucchini and squash noodles in a colander in the sink and sprinkle with ¼ teaspoon salt. Let sit for at least 20 minutes before rinsing the noodles and letting dry briefly.

2.   Add the cashews, lemon juice, water, olive oil, turmeric, garlic, onion powder, nutritional yeast, 1 teaspoon salt and pepper to a blender or food processor. Blend until smooth, adding more water if necessary.

3.   In a serving bowl combine the noodles, cherry tomatoes and the cashew mixture. Garnish with chives.

Butternut Squash Risotto

Servings: 2

Total Time: 1 hour 10 minutes

Ingredients

- 1 cup butternut squash, peeled, seeded and cut into small cubes

- 1 teaspoon olive oil

- 3 cups vegetable broth

- 1 tablespoon ghee

- ½ yellow onion, diced

- ½ bunch kale, stems removed and cut into thin ribbons

- 4 fresh sage leaves, thinly sliced

- ½ teaspoon Himalayan pink salt

- ¼ teaspoon freshly ground pepper

- ½ cup brown rice

- 1 cup butternut squash, peeled, seeded and cut into small cubes

- 1 cup brown rice

- 1 tablespoon chives, thinly sliced

Directions

1.   Roast butternut squash in an oven preheated to 400°F/205°C by lining squash cubes on a baking tray lined with parchment paper and drizzling squash with 1 teaspoon olive oil. Roast for 25 minutes, flipping once.

2.   In a small saucepan, bring broth to a low simmer over low heat.

3.   Place ghee in a large saucepan over medium-low heat and add onion, kale, sage salt and pepper. Cook 5 minutes before adding brown rice and cooking another 2 minutes to toast.

4.   Add butternut squash and brown rice to the large saucepan before adding a ¼ cup of the broth and stirring. Reduce heat to low. Continue adding ¼ cup broth and stirring once the previously adding liquid has been absorbed. This may take up to 50 minutes.

5.   Remove risotto and place in serving bowl and garnish with chives.

Meatless Meatloaf Cups

Servings: 2 (3 cups per serving)

Total Time: 1 hour 10 minutes

Ingredients

- 1 tablespoon of ground flaxseeds + 3 ½ tablespoons of water

- 1 ½ tablespoon olive oil

- 1 small carrot, peeled and cut into 1 inch pieces

- 1 small celery stalk, cut into 1 inch pieces

- 1 shallot, diced

- 1 garlic clove, minced

- ½ cup button mushrooms, diced

- 1 cup brown lentils, cooked

- ¼ cup walnuts, toasted

- ½ cup almond meal

- 1 teaspoon Dijon mustard

- 1 teaspoon paprika

- 1 teaspoon Himalayan salt

- 1 teaspoon black pepper

- ½ tablespoon olive oil

- 1 tablespoon tomato paste

- 1 teaspoon raw honey

- 1 teaspoon coconut aminos

- 1 teaspoon tamari

Directions

1. In a small bowl, whisk to combine the flaxseeds and water. Set aside.

2. Heat 1 tablespoon olive oil in a medium skillet over medium-low heat. Add carrot, celery, shallots and garlic. Cook 10 minutes, stirring frequently. Add mushrooms and cook another 10 minutes.

3. Place lentils and walnuts in food processor and pulse together about 10 times. Add vegetable mixture to the food processor and mix until combined but not entirely smooth. Add mixture to a bowl and fold in the almond meal, flaxseeds mixture, mustard, paprika, salt and pepper.

4. Lightly grease 6 places in a muffin tin with ½ tablespoon olive oil. Add lentil and vegetable mixture to each and press to mold.

5.   In a small bowl, combine tomato paste, honey, coconut aminos and tamari. Brush tomato mixture on top of each meatloaf cup.

6.   Bake in an oven that has been preheated to 350°F/180°C for 40 minutes. Tops should be lightly browned when finished.

Spicy Dal & Greens

Servings: 2

Total Time: 30 minutes

Ingredients

- 1 tablespoon ghee
- 1 jalapeno, seeded and diced
- ¼ teaspoon ground cumin
- ¼ teaspoon turmeric
- ¼ teaspoon ground cardamom
- ⅛ teaspoon ground fenugreek
- 1 inch piece ginger, grated
- 1 garlic clove, minced
- 1 small onion, diced
- 1 small tomato, diced
- ½ cup red lentils, rinsed and drained
- 1 cup vegetable broth
- ¼ teaspoon Himalayan salt
- 1 teaspoon black pepper, crushed
- 2 tablespoons cilantro, chopped

- 1 lime, zest

Directions

1.   Heat ghee in a medium saucepan over medium high heat. Add jalapeno, cumin, turmeric, cardamom, fenugreek, ginger, garlic and onion. Cook 5 minutes and then add tomato and red lentils. Stir and cook for an additional minute.

2.   Pour vegetable broth into the saucepan and add salt and pepper. Bring to a boil and then reduce heat to low and simmer about 15 - 20 minutes or until lentils are soft.

3.   Garnish with cilantro and lime zest.

Blackened Salmon with Fruit Salsa

Servings: 2

Total Time: 20 minutes

Ingredients

- 8 ounces wild salmon fillet, skin-on
- 1 teaspoon cayenne pepper
- 1 teaspoon garlic powder
- ½ teaspoon chili powder
- ¼ teaspoon Himalayan salt
- ¼ teaspoon black pepper, crushed
- 1 tablespoon olive oil
- 4 cups mixed greens (e.g. spring onions, broccoli, spinach)

Mango Pineapple Salsa

- ½ green bell pepper, seeded and diced into small pieces
- ½ cup mango, diced into small pieces
- ½ cup pineapple, diced into small pieces
- 1 lime, zested and juiced
- 1 tablespoon cilantro, finely chopped
- Pinch Himalayan salt

Directions

1. Make the Mango Pineapple Salsa by placing all the Mango Pineapple Salsa ingredients in a small bowl and combining well. Set aside.

2. In a small bowl, combine the cayenne, garlic powder, chili powder, salt and pepper. Place mixture on flat plate.

3. Heat a cast iron skillet on the stovetop over medium heat. Brush the olive oil on each side of each fillet and then place the flesh side in the spice mixture on the plate.

4. Place the fish, flesh side down in the pan and cook about 5 minutes. Flip over cook an additional 6 minutes or until fish is done.

5. Serve fish over mixed greens (of your liking) and spoon salsa on top.

Roasted Cauliflower with Chimichurri Sauce

Servings: 2

Total Time: 40 minutes

Ingredients

- 1 small head cauliflower (about 1 pound), stem removed

- 2 tablespoons avocado oil, divided

- 1 teaspoon Himalayan salt, divided

- 1 teaspoon dried oregano

- ½ teaspoon black pepper

- 2 garlic cloves, minced and divided

- 3 cups green beans, trimmed

- 15 cherry tomatoes, halved

- 1 teaspoon lemon zest

Chimichurri Sauce

- ¼ cup apple cider vinegar

- ½ teaspoon Himalayan salt

- 2 garlic cloves

- 1 shallot, sliced

- 1 teaspoon red chili flakes

- 1 teaspoon fresh oregano (or dried)

- ¼ cup cilantro, chopped

- ¼ cup flat-leaf parsley, chopped

- 1/3 cup olive oil

Directions

1.   Make Chimichurri Sauce by placing all ingredients except the olive oil in a food processor or blender and blend until combined. While the food processor is running, drizzle in the olive oil. Let it sit while preparing the cauliflower.

2.   Slice the cauliflower in half lengthwise and cut two steaks from each side of the core (saving any leftover cauliflower that falls loose).

3.   Heat a large cast iron skillet (or ovenproof skillet) on the stove over medium-high heat. Add 1 tablespoon of the avocado oil and once heated, place cauliflower steaks into the skillet. Season with 1/4 teaspoon salt, ½ teaspoon oregano and ¼ teaspoon black pepper. After 4 minutes, flip and season the other side with ¼ teaspoon salt, ½ teaspoon oregano and ¼ teaspoon black pepper. Cook for another 4 minutes before placing pan in an oven that has been preheated to 400°F/205°C. Roast for 20 minutes or until cauliflower is tender.

4.   On a baking tray lined with parchment paper, place the green beans and tomatoes. Drizzle with remaining olive oil and sprinkle salt, pepper, garlic and lemon zest on top. Roast in the oven with the cauliflower for 15 minutes, turning once.

5.   Serve cauliflower on top of the green bean/tomato mixture and drizzled with Chimichurri Sauce.

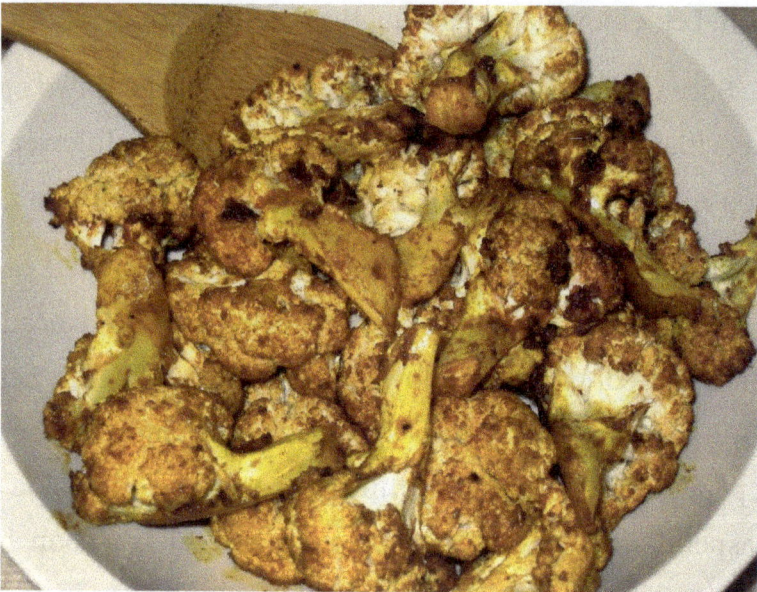

Cook-off Chili

Servings: 2

Total Time: 20 minutes

Ingredients

- 1 tablespoon olive oil
- ½ small onion, diced
- 1 jalapeno pepper, seeded and diced
- 1 small carrot, diced
- ½ red bell pepper, seeded and diced
- 1 small tomato, diced
- 1 tablespoon tomato paste
- 2 garlic cloves, minced
- 1 ½ teaspoon chili powder
- 1 ½ teaspoon cumin powder
- ½ cup cooked red beans
- ½ cup quinoa, cooked
- 2 cups vegetable stock
- 1 lime, sliced in half
- 2 tablespoons cilantro, chopped

- 2 tablespoons unsweetened yogurt

Directions

1.   In a large pot over medium heat, add olive oil, onion, jalapeno, carrot and red bell pepper. Cook 8 minutes or until softened. Add in tomatoes, tomato paste, garlic, chili powder, cumin, red beans, quinoa and vegetable stock.

2.   Bring to a boil, reduce heat to low and simmer 15 minutes.

3.   Serve in two bowls and garnish each bowl with ½ lime, 1 tablespoon cilantro and 1 tablespoon yogurt each.

Pasta & Veggie Stroganoff

Servings: 2

Total Time: 20 minutes

Ingredients

- 8 ounces gluten-free pasta

- 1 tablespoon olive oil

- 1 garlic clove, minced

- 1 cup mushrooms, sliced

- 2 cups spinach

- 1 teaspoon red pepper flakes

- 1 teaspoon oregano

- ½ teaspoon nutmeg

- 1 cup unsweetened almond milk

- 1 cup vegetable broth

- 1 teaspoon arrowroot starch

- ¼ teaspoon Himalayan salt

- ½ teaspoon black pepper, crushed

- ¼ cup parsley, chopped

Directions

1.   Cook pasta according to package directions.

2.   In a large skillet over medium heat, add olive oil, garlic and mushrooms. Cook 5 minutes then add spinach, red pepper, oregano, nutmeg and cook 3 more minutes.

3.   Pour in almond milk and vegetable broth. Sprinkle the arrowroot starch on top and stir well. Let come to a low boil then reduce heat to a simmer and cook 5 minutes. Season with salt and pepper.

4.   Place pasta on a plate and top with mushroom spinach mixture. Garnish with chopped parsley.

Tofu Mole with Jicama Salad

Servings: 2

Total Time: 35 minutes

Ingredients

- 4 cups kale, stems removed and sliced into thin ribbons
- 1 tablespoon olive oil
- 1 lemon, juiced
- ½ teaspoon Himalayan salt
- 8 ounces firm tofu, cubed and baked
- 1 cup jicama, peeled and shredded
- 1 tablespoon raisins
- 1 teaspoon slivered almonds

Mole Sauce

- 1 tablespoon olive oil
- ½ onion, chopped
- 1 garlic clove, minced
- 1/3 cup slivered almonds
- ¼ cup raisins
- 3 dates, pitted, soaked 15 minutes and drained

- ½ teaspoon Himalayan salt

- ¼ teaspoon cinnamon

- ½ teaspoon ground coriander

- 1 teaspoon cumin

- 1 teaspoon dried thyme

- 1 teaspoon chili powder

- ¼ teaspoon ground cloves

- 1 teaspoon chipotle in adobo sauce

- 1 tablespoon tomato paste

- ¼ cup diced tomatoes

- ½ cup water

- 1 tablespoon raw cacao

Directions

1. Place kale in a large bowl and add in olive oil. Massage gently then add lemon juice and salt. Set aside while making Mole Sauce.

2. Make Mole Sauce by heating olive oil in a large saucepan over medium heat. Add the onion, garlic, almonds, raisins and dates. Cook for 8 minutes. Stir in the salt, cinnamon, coriander, cumin, thyme, chili powder and cloves. Cook 1 minute.

3.   Add chipotle, tomato paste, tomatoes, water and cacao to the saucepan and simmer for 15 minutes. Turn heat off and blend with immersion blender (or let cool and blend in a blender).

4.   Add Mole Sauce back to the saucepan and add baked tofu. Turn heat to low and allow to heat through.

5.   Toss jicama, raisins and almonds in the kale mixture and place on a plate along with the tofu mole.

Green Pea Pasta

Servings: 2

Total Time: 35 minutes

Ingredients

- ½ tablespoon olive oil
- 1 garlic clove, minced
- 1 ½ tablespoons ginger, peeled and grated
- 2 cups spinach
- 1 cup coconut milk
- 1 tablespoon lime juice
- ½ teaspoon red chili flakes
- ½ cup cilantro
- ½ cup green peas, defrosted
- 2 medium zucchinis, spiralized into noodles
- 1 teaspoon Himalayan salt
- 1 teaspoon black pepper

Directions

1. Heat oil in a medium skillet over medium heat. Add garlic and ginger and cook 3 minutes. Add spinach, coconut milk, lime juice, chili flakes and cilantro. Simmer for 5 minutes.

2. Add mixture to a high speed blender along with ¼ cup green peas. Blend until smooth to create the saucy mixture.

3. Place medium skillet back over medium heat and add zucchini noodles, remaining ¼ cup peas and sauce. Heat for 3 minutes and sprinkle salt and pepper before serving.

Tricolor Pasta

Servings: 2

Total Time: 20 minutes

Ingredients

- 2 medium beets, spiralized into noodles
- 1 tablespoon olive oil
- ½ teaspoon Himalayan salt

Green Sauce

- 1 cup basil leaves, packed
- 1 cup parsley, chopped
- ½ cup spinach, chopped
- 3 tablespoons almonds
- 1 tablespoon green onion, chopped
- ¼ cup of olive oil
- ½ teaspoon Himalayan salt
- ¼ teaspoon black pepper, crushed
- 1 large clove
- 1 teaspoon cayenne

Spicy Orange Garnish

- 1 small carrot, shredded

- 1 tablespoon olive oil

- 1 teaspoon red chili flakes

- 1 teaspoon pumpkin seeds, toasted

- ¼ teaspoon turmeric

- 1 teaspoon lemon juice

Directions

1. Line a baking tray with parchment paper. Coat beet noodles with tablespoon of olive oil and spread on the baking tray. Season with ½ teaspoon salt.

2. Bake in an oven preheated to 400°F/205°C for 15 minutes.

3. In a small bowl, combine ingredients for the Spicy Orange Garnish and set aside.

4. In a food processor or blender, combine all the Green Sauce ingredients and mix until smooth.

5. Remove beet noodles from oven, place in a large bowl and toss with Green Sauce. Top with Spicy Orange Garnish.

Cauliflower Pasta Pillows in Red Sauce

Servings: 2

Total Time: 45 minutes

Ingredients

- 1 head of cauliflower, steamed

- 1 garlic clove, minced

- 1 cup almond meal of enough to make a soft dough

- ¼ cup arrowroot powder (plus extra for rolling out dough)

- 1 tablespoon ground flaxseeds

- 3 tablespoons water

- 1 tablespoon olive oil

- ½ cup basil leaves, thinly sliced

Red Sauce

- ½ onion, chopped

- 1 tablespoon olive oil

- 1 garlic clove, minced

- 1 small carrot, chopped

- 1 red bell pepper, chopped

- 1 cup cherry tomatoes, halved

- 1 ½ cups vegetable stock

- 1 teaspoon oregano

- 1 teaspoon dried basil

- 1 teaspoon Himalayan salt

- 1 teaspoon pepper

Directions

1.   Whisk together the flaxseeds and water together in a small bowl. Set aside.

2.   *For creation of the Red Sauce* In a medium skillet over medium heat, add onion, olive oil, garlic, carrot and red pepper. Cook 10 minutes and then add tomatoes, vegetable stock, oregano, dried basil, salt and pepper. Cook another 10 minutes.

3.   Using an immersion blender, blend the Red Sauce until smooth. Reduce heat to low and simmer another 20 minutes while you make the cauliflower pasta.

4.   In a food processor, add the cauliflower and garlic. Process until smooth. In a small bowl combine the almond meal, arrowroot powder and flaxseeds mixture (it should now be a gel). Add to the food processor in small increments, blending between each addition. If needed, add some water to make a soft dough.

5.   Dust cutting board with extra arrowroot powder and place dough on the board. Roll the dough into 4 equal sized ropes. Cut the ropes into 1 inch pieces. Press each piece lightly with a fork.

6.   In a medium skillet, heat olive oil over medium-low heat. Add cauliflower pasta pieces, making sure not to crowd the pan and cook 3 minutes each side.

7.   Place cauliflower pasta on a place and top with Red Sauce and basil leaves.

Raw Thai Curry

Servings: 2

Total Time: 10 minutes

Ingredients

- 2 medium yellow squash, spiralized into noodles
- ½ cup alfalfa sprouts
- ¼ cup green peas, defrosted
- 1 red pepper, sliced
- ¼ red cabbage, shredded
- ¼ cup cilantro, chopped
- 2 tablespoons cashews, toasted and crushed
- 2 tablespoons green onions, thinly sliced

Curry Sauce

- 1 tablespoon green curry paste
- ½ cup raw cashew nuts, soaked for 30 minutes and drained
- ¼ cup water
- ½ lime, juiced
- 2 tablespoons cilantro, chopped

- ¼ cup green onion, chopped

- ¼ cup coconut milk

- ½ teaspoon ground cumin

- ½ teaspoon ground ginger

- 1 garlic clove, minced

- ½ inch piece fresh ginger, grated

- ½ teaspoon ground coriander

- 1 teaspoon red chili flakes

Directions

1.   In a high speed blender, add Curry Sauce ingredients and blend until smooth.

2.   Toss together the squash, sprouts, green peas, bell pepper, cabbage and cilantro. Add Curry Sauce and toss to coat well. Garnish with cashews and green onions.

Shrimp & Arugula Salad

Servings: 2

Total Time: 25 minutes

Ingredients

- 10 large shrimp, peeled, cleaned and deveined
- ½ lemon, juiced
- 2 tablespoons olive oil
- 1 garlic clove, minced
- 1 tablespoon parsley, chopped
- ½ teaspoon Himalayan salt
- ½ teaspoon black pepper, crushed

Arugula Salad

- 4 cups arugula
- 10 cherry tomatoes, halved
- 2 tablespoons apple cider vinegar
- ½ lemon, juiced
- 2 tablespoons olive oil
- 1 teaspoon Himalayan salt
- 2 teaspoons pine nuts, toasted

Directions

1.   In a medium bowl, place shrimp, lemon juice, olive oil, garlic, parsley, salt and pepper. Let sit in the fridge for 15 minutes.

2.   Heat a medium skillet or grill pan over medium-high heat. Place shrimp in the skillet and cook 3 minutes each side or until shrimp are pink and firm.

3.   Combine the ingredients for the Arugula Salad in a large bowl. Place shrimp on top of the salad and serve.

Avocado and Tomato Pizza

Servings: 2

Total Time: 15 minutes plus 12 hours dehydrating time

Ingredients

- 1 avocado, sliced

- 1 small tomato, sliced

- 1 cup arugula

- 2 teaspoons olive oil

- 2 tablespoons nutritional yeast

- 1 teaspoon Himalayan salt

- 1 teaspoon lemon juice

Pizza Dough

- 1 ¼ cups sunflower seeds, soaked overnight and drained

- 1/3 cup flaxseeds, ground to a very fine powder

- 1 garlic clove, minced

- 4 tablespoons olive oil

- 1 teaspoon Himalayan salt

- 1 teaspoon black pepper, crushed

- 1 teaspoon dried oregano

- 1 teaspoon dried basil

Directions

1.   In a blender, pulse the drained sunflower seeds a few times then add sunflower mix to a medium bowl along with the flaxseeds flour, garlic, olive oil, salt, pepper, oregano and basil.

2.   Knead together the mixture until a dough forms (add a little water if needed). Roll out dough into a pizza shape and place on a baking tray lined with parchment paper.

3.   Heat oven to lowest possible temperature. Place baking tray in the oven and dehydrate in the oven for at least 12 hours.

4.   When Pizza Dough is ready, layer avocado and tomato slices on top of the crust. Toss arugula in a small bowl with olive oil, nutritional yeast, salt and lemon juice. Place arugula on top of avocado and tomato. Serve immediately.

Spinach Ravioli

Servings: 2

Total Time: 1 hour

Ingredients

- 1 tablespoon flaxseed, ground

- 6 tablespoons water, divided

- 1 cup spelt flour

- 1 teaspoon Himalayan salt

Spinach Filling

- 1 tablespoon flaxseed, ground

- 3 tablespoons water

- ½ cup mushrooms, sliced

- 1 cup spinach

- 1 teaspoon olive oil

- 1 tablespoon parsley, chopped

- 1 tablespoon nutritional yeast

Simple Red Sauce

- 1 cup cherry tomatoes, halved

- 1 red bell pepper, chopped

- 2 tablespoons olive oil

- 1 clove garlic, grated

- ½ cup water

- 1 teaspoon oregano

- 1 teaspoon Himalayan salt

- 1 teaspoon pepper

Directions

1. Make the spinach filling by whisking together the ground flaxseeds and water together in a small bowl and letting sit for 15 minutes. After 15 minutes, add flax mixture and remaining Spinach Filling ingredients to a food processor and combine. Set aside.

2. Prepare Simple Red Sauce by combining all Simple Red Sauce ingredients in a blender and combining until smooth.

3. To make ravioli, begin by creating a flask egg by whisking together 1 tablespoon flaxseeds with 3 tablespoons water and letting rest 15 minutes. When ready, combine flax mixture, spelt flour, salt and remaining 3 tablespoons water in a food processor until a dough forms. Let dough rest for 20 minutes.

4. Roll out dough and use a ravioli maker to fill each with the Spinach Filling and top with second layer of dough. Seal edges with water.

5.   Boil water in a medium saucepan and once at a rolling boil, drop in ravioli and cook 6 minutes. Strain and set aside.

6.   Add Simple Red Sauce to medium saucepan and bring to a simmer. Add ravioli and cook 2 minutes until warmed.

Kale & Squash Vegetable Gratin

Servings: 2

Total Time: 50 minutes

Ingredients

- 2 tablespoons ghee

- 1 garlic clove, finely minced

- 1 leek, finely chopped

- 1 fennel bulb, sliced

- 2 cups kale, stems removed and thinly sliced

- 2 cups butternut squash, cubed and roasted

- ¼ cup rice flour

- ½ cup unsweetened almond milk, warmed

- 1 teaspoon dried sage

- ½ teaspoon nutmeg

- 1 teaspoon Himalayan salt

- 1 teaspoon black pepper, crushed

Crumb Topping

- 1 ½ tablespoons ghee

- 1 cup gluten-free oats

- ¼ cup almond meal

- ¼ cup almonds, slivered

- 1 teaspoon fresh sage, torn

- 1 teaspoon Himalayan salt

Directions

1. Prepare vegetable filling by heating 1 tablespoon ghee in a medium saucepan over medium heat. Add garlic, leek and fennel. Cook 10 minutes and then add kale. Cook another 5 minutes and then transfer to a small baking dish. Place roasted butternut squash on top of the vegetable mixture.

2. Make the sauce by adding 1 tablespoon ghee to the medium saucepan and heat over medium-low heat. When ghee is melted, whisk in rice flour and continue to move around the pan about 5 minutes. Pour in warmed almond milk while continuing to whisk. Bring to a boil, then reduce heat to low and simmer. Season with sage, nutmeg, salt and pepper.

3. Pour sauce over the vegetable and squash mixture, making sure it is well combined. Preheat oven to 325°F/170°C.

4. To make the Crumb Topping, melt 1 ½ tablespoons ghee in a large skillet. Then add remaining Crumb Topping ingredients. Let cool slightly and then crumble the mixture on top of the vegetable and squash mixture.

5.   Bake in the oven for 30 minutes. Serve immediately from the oven.

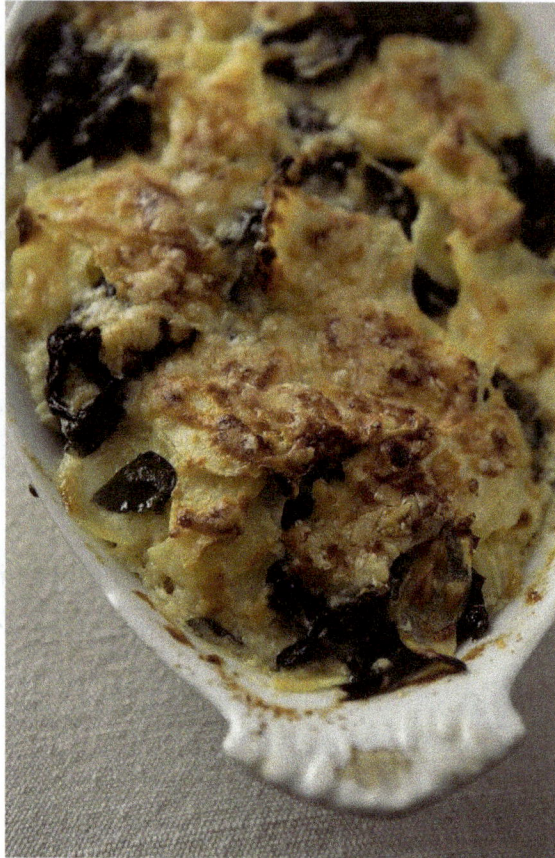

Spicy Orange Sweet Potato Bowl

Servings: 1

Total Time: 40 minutes

Ingredients

- 1 medium sweet potato, cubed

- 2 teaspoons sesame seed oil

- 1 date, pitted and soaked 10 minutes and drained

- 3 tablespoon orange juice

- 1 tablespoon tamari

- 1 tablespoon coconut aminos

- 1 garlic clove, grated

- ½ teaspoon red chili flakes

- ½ teaspoon ginger, grated

- 2 cups broccoli, cut into florets, steamed

- 1 tablespoon sesame seeds

Directions

1.   Preheat oven to 400°F/205°C and place sweet potato on a baking tray lined with parchment paper. Coat sweet potato with 1 teaspoon sesame seed oil and then bake in the oven for 30 minutes.

2.   In a blender, combine the date, orange juice, tamari, coconut aminos, garlic, red chili flakes and ginger. Set aside.

3.   In a medium skillet, heat remaining sesame oil over medium-low and add steamed broccoli. Cook 3 minutes and set aside.

4.   Add orange juice mixture to the pan and let come to a low simmer. Add the sweet potato and toss to coat. Cook 5 minutes until sauce is reduced slightly.

5.   Serve sweet potato alongside the broccoli and garnish with sesame seeds.

Cauliflower Colcannon

Servings: 2

Total Time: 5 minutes

Ingredients

- 1 cauliflower, cut into florets and steamed

- ½ cup parsley, chopped

- 1 garlic clove, chopped

- 1 tablespoon lemon juice

- 2 tablespoon olive oil

- ½ teaspoon Himalayan salt

- 1 cup brussel sprouts, shredded

- 1 cup green cabbage, thinly shredded

- 1 tablespoon green onions, sliced

Directions

1.   Place steamed cauliflower, parsley, garlic clove, lemon juice, olive oil and salt in a food processor and blend until smooth.

2.   Add the brussel sprouts and cabbage to the food processor and pulse 3-4 times so that the sprouts and cabbage are incorporated but not completely pureed.

3.   Transfer to a bowl and garnish with green onion.

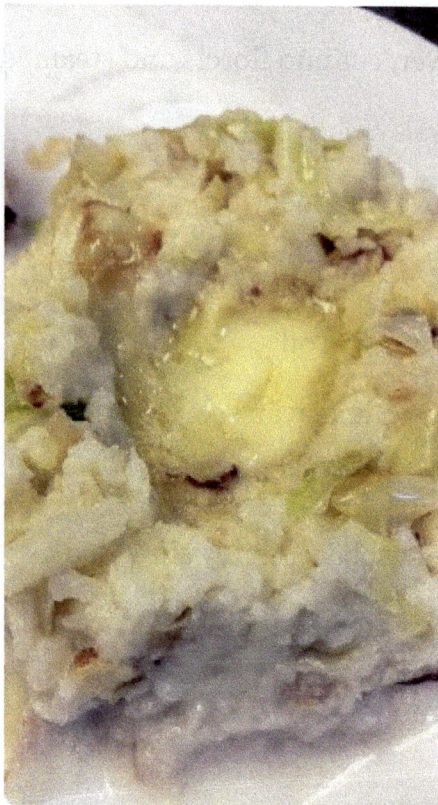

Peas & Rice

Servings: 2

Total Time: 10 minutes

Ingredients

- 3 tablespoons coconut oil
- 2 red chilies, chopped
- 2 garlic cloves, chopped
- ½ teaspoon fresh ginger, grated
- 1 shallot, sliced
- 1 pound green beans
- 3 tablespoons coconut milk
- 1 tablespoon unsweetened, shredded coconut
- ½ teaspoon Himalayan salt
- ½ teaspoon cayenne pepper
- 1 cup brown rice, cooked

Directions

1.   In a medium sized skillet over medium heat add coconut oil, chilies, garlic, ginger and shallots. Cook for 5 minutes and

then add green beans, coconut milk, shredded coconut, salt and pepper.

2.   Reduce heat to low and cook 5 minutes.

3.   Serve on top of brown rice.

Sweet & Spicy Sweet Potato Skillet

Servings: 2

Total Time: 25 minutes

Ingredients

- 1 tablespoon olive oil

- ½ red onion, sliced

- 2 sweet potatoes, cubed

- ½ teaspoon cayenne pepper

- ½ teaspoon red chili flakes

- ½ teaspoon cumin

- ½ teaspoon Himalayan salt

- ½ teaspoon black pepper, crushed

- 1 apple, cored and cubed

- 1 cup chickpeas, cooked

- ½ cup quinoa, cooked

- ¼ cup walnuts, toasted and crushed

- 1 teaspoon raw honey

- 2 tablespoons cilantro, chopped

Directions

1.   Heat oil in a medium skillet over medium-high heat and add onions. Cook 5 minutes and then add sweet potato, cayenne, chili flakes, cumin, salt and pepper.

2.   Cook for 15 minutes until tender and crispy, stirring frequently.

3.   Add in apple and cook 2 minutes and then add chickpeas, quinoa, walnuts and honey.

4.   Garnish with cilantro and serve warm.

Broccoli & Pear Salad

Servings: 2

Total Time: 20 minutes

Ingredients

- 1 head of broccoli, shredded into very small florets
- 1 pear, cored and chopped
- ¼ red onion, thinly sliced
- 2 tablespoons cup walnuts, crushed
- 2 tablespoons cup pepitas
- ¼ cup raisins

Dressing

- ¾ cup unsweetened yogurt
- 2 tablespoons apple cider vinegar
- 1 tablespoon lemon juice
- 1 tablespoon honey
- ¼ teaspoon Himalayan salt

Directions

1. In a large bowl, combine the broccoli, pear, red onion, walnuts, pepitas and raisins.

2. Whisk together the Dressing ingredients in a small bowl and pour over broccoli mixture.

3. Toss well to coat and let sit in the fridge for 10 minutes before serving.

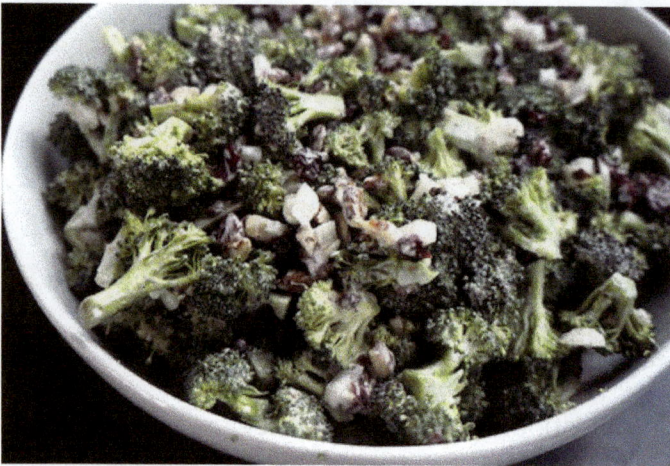

Quinoa Niçoise Salad

Servings: 1

Total Time: 10 minutes

Ingredients

- 2 cups kale, stems removed and thinly sliced
- 1 teaspoon lemon juice
- ½ cup quinoa, cooked
- 1 cup green beans, cut in half and steamed
- ¼ cup black olives, sliced
- ½ cup sweet potato, diced and steamed
- 1 small tomato, diced
- 1 tablespoon olive oil
- ¼ teaspoon Himalayan salt
- ¼ teaspoon black pepper, crushed

Directions

1. Place kale in a large bowl and add lemon juice. Gently massage the kale and then let sit for 5 minutes.

2. After 5 minutes, place kale on a large plate and top with quinoa, green beans, olives, sweet potato and tomato.

3. Drizzle with olive oil and season with salt and pepper.

Red & Green Salad

Servings: 1

Total Time: 10 minutes

Ingredients

- 1 cup quinoa, cooked
- 2 cups fresh baby spinach, chopped
- 2 cups arugula
- 1 pint strawberries, hulled and sliced
- 1 avocado, diced
- ¼ cup pepitas, toasted
- 1 shallot, thinly sliced

Dressing

- 1/2 cup avocado oil
- 3 tablespoons apple cider vinegar
- 1 tablespoon honey
- ½ teaspoon Himalayan salt
- ½ teaspoon black pepper, crushed

Directions

1.   In a small bowl, whisk together the Dressing ingredients and set aside.

2.   Combine quinoa, spinach, arugula, strawberries, avocado, pepitas and shallot in a large bowl.

3.   Pour dressing over and toss well to coat.

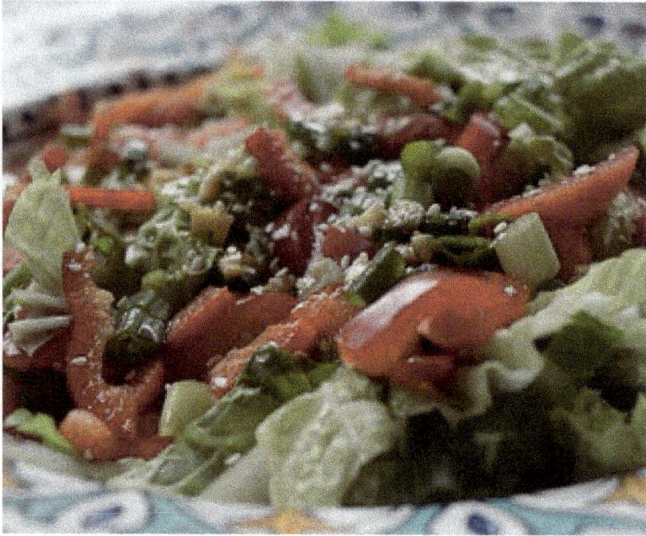

Shredded Kale Salad

Servings: 2

Total Time: 5 minutes

Ingredients

- 1 cup brussel sprouts, finely shredded
- 1 cup kale, stems removed and finely chopped
- 1 cup red cabbage, finely shredded
- ¼ cup wild rice, cooked
- ¼ cup almonds
- ¼ cup pomegranate seeds
- 1 tablespoon olive oil
- 1 lime, juiced
- 2 teaspoons apple cider vinegar
- 1 teaspoon honey
- ½ teaspoon Himalayan salt
- ¼ teaspoon black pepper

Directions

1. Combine all ingredients in a large bowl and toss to coat well.

2. Serve immediately.

Italian Kale Stew

Servings: 2

Total Time: 30 minutes

Ingredients

- 1 tablespoon olive oil
- ½ medium onion, finely diced
- 2 garlic cloves, chopped
- 1 teaspoon dried oregano
- ½ teaspoon dried thyme
- 1 ½ cups chickpeas, cooked
- 1 tomato, diced
- 1 tablespoon tomato paste
- 3 cups vegetable broth
- 3 cups kale, stems removed and finely chopped
- ¼ cup fresh parsley, chopped
- ½ teaspoon Himalayan salt

Directions

1.   Heat oil in a large pot over medium heat. Add onion, garlic, oregano and thyme. Cook 7 minutes.

2.   Add chickpeas, tomato, tomato paste and vegetable broth. Bring to a boil and then reduce heat to a simmer and cook for 20 minutes.

3.   Stir in kale and let it wilt before stirring in parsley and salt.

4.   Serve immediately.

Spinach & Beet Salad

Servings: 2

Total Time: 5 minutes

Ingredients

- 4 cups spinach, chopped
- ½ cup fresh parsley, chopped
- 1 cup quinoa, cooked
- 1 cup beets, cooked and grated
- 1 cup lentils, cooked

Dressing

- 1 lemon, juiced
- 2 tablespoons tahini
- 1 tablespoon warm water
- ½ teaspoon Himalayan salt
- ½ teaspoon black pepper

Directions

1. In a small bowl, whisk together the Dressing ingredients.

2.   Place spinach, parsley, quinoa, beets and lentils in a large bowl and pour in the Dressing.

3.   Toss well to coat and serve immediately.

Spicy Cabbage Bowl

Servings: 2

Total Time: 10 minutes

Ingredients

- 2 teaspoons sesame oil
- ½ teaspoon fresh ginger, grated
- 1 teaspoon garlic, minced
- 1 cup brown rice, cooked
- 1 cup cabbage kimchi, chopped
- 2 teaspoons tamari
- 1 teaspoon coconut aminos
- 2 cups kale, stems removed and finely chopped
- ¼ cup green onion
- 1 tablespoon sesame seeds

Directions

1.   Heat sesame oil in a medium skillet over medium heat and add ginger, garlic, brown rice, kimchi, tamari and coconut aminos.

2.   Let cook 5 minutes and then add in the kale and green onions. Toss well to combine and cook 4 minutes.

3.   Garnish with sesame seeds before serving.

Fennel Citrus Salad

Servings: 2

Total Time: 10 minutes

Ingredients

- 1 small orange, segmented
- ½ small red grapefruit, segmented
- 2 small fennel bulbs, thinly sliced
- ½ cup parsley, chopped
- 1 tablespoon mint, chopped
- 2 tablespoons fresh lemon juice
- 2 tablespoons fresh orange juice
- ¼ cup olive oil
- ⅛ teaspoon sea salt
- ½ teaspoon freshly ground black pepper
- 2 tablespoons pomegranate seeds
- ½ avocado, diced

Directions

1.　　In a large bowl, combine the orange segments, grapefruit segments, fennel slices, mint and parsley.

2.　　Whisk together lemon juice, orange juice, olive oil, salt and pepper. Pour over the citrus and fennel mixture. Toss well to coat.

3.　　Transfer to plate and garnish with pomegranate seeds and avocado. Serve immediately.

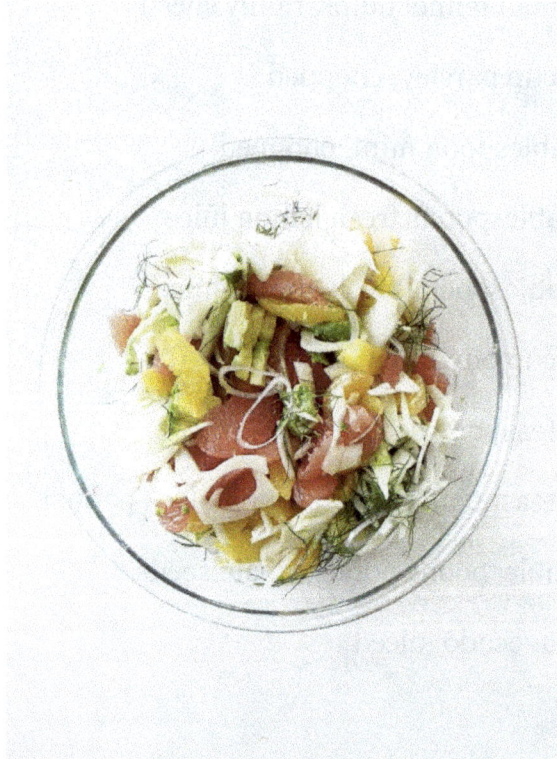

Salmon & Vegetable Kebabs with Greens Pesto

Servings: 2

Total Time: 30 minutes

Ingredients

- 6 ounces wild, fresh salmon, skin removed and cut into 1 inch cubes

- 1 small zucchini, chopped into 1 inch pieces

- 12 cherry tomatoes

- 1 small yellow pepper, cut into 1 inch pieces

- ½ sweet onion, quartered and divided into 12 pieces

- 1 tablespoon olive oil

- 1 garlic clove, minced

- ½ teaspoon Himalayan salt

- ¼ teaspoon black pepper, crushed

- 4 wooden skewers, soaked in water for at least 30 minutes

Pesto Sauce

- 1 cup spinach

- 1 garlic clove, minced

- ½ cup basil leaves

- ¼ cup pumpkin seeds

- ¼ cup olive oil

- 1 teaspoon Himalayan salt

- ½ teaspoon pepper

- 1 lemon, juiced

Directions

1. Thread salmon and vegetables on skewers in desired pattern. Place skewers on a baking tray. Brush kebabs with olive oil, garlic, salt and pepper.

2. Place skewers in an oven that has been preheated to 400°F/205°C and bake for approximately 20 minutes, turning once and making sure fish is cooked through.

3. In a blender or food processor, place the ingredients for the Pesto Sauce and combine until smooth, adding more olive oil if too thick. Drizzle over cooked skewers.

Coconut Curry & Vegetables

Servings: 2

Total Time: 25 minutes

Ingredients

- 2 tablespoons coconut oil
- ½ yellow onion, diced
- 1 teaspoon fresh ginger, grated
- 2 medium zucchinis, cubed into 1 inch pieces
- 1 yellow bell pepper, cut into 1 inch pieces
- ½ cup eggplant, cubed into 1 inch pieces
- ¼ pound green beans, cut into 1 inch pieces
- 8 ounces firm tofu, cut into 1 inch pieces
- 1 tomato, diced
- 1 cup coconut milk
- 1/3 cup water
- 1 teaspoon Himalayan salt
- 2 teaspoons curry powder
- 3 tablespoons cilantro, chopped

Directions

1.   In a medium skillet heat coconut oil and add onion, ginger, zucchini, bell pepper, eggplant and beans. Cook for 5 minutes before adding the tofu and tomatoes. Let sauté for another 5 minutes.

2.   Add coconut milk, water, salt, and curry powder. Let simmer 10 minutes. Stir in cilantro before serving.

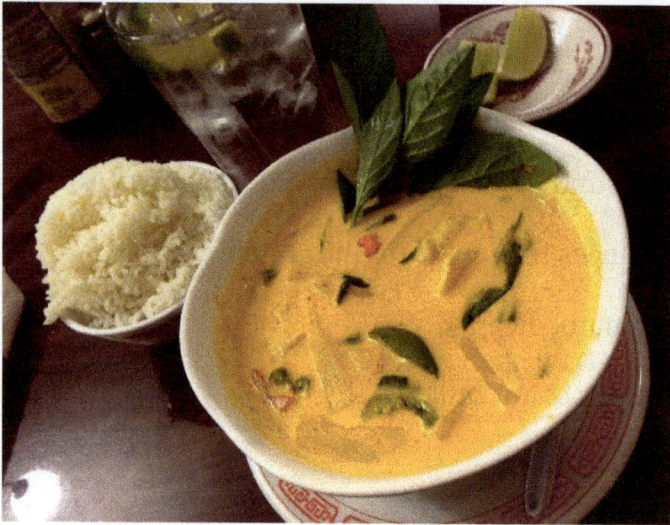

Loaded Spaghetti Squash

Servings: 2

Total Time: 40 minutes

Ingredients

- 1 spaghetti squash, cut in half lengthwise and seeds removed

- 1 ½ tablespoons olive oil

- 1 leek, chopped

- 1 garlic clove, minced

- 6 tomatoes, diced

- 1 cup cooked green or brown lentils

- ½ teaspoon oregano

- ½ teaspoon Himalayan salt

- 1 cup basil leaves, torn

- ½ teaspoon lemon zest

Directions

1. Rub 1 tablespoon of the olive oil on each of the spaghetti squash halves and place face down on a baking tray lined with

parchment paper. Place in a 375°F/190°C oven for 30 minutes or until squash are tender.

2.   In a skillet, heat remaining ½ tablespoon olive oil and add the leek, garlic and tomatoes. Cook 8 minutes before adding in the lentils and dried oregano. Continue to cook for another 5 minutes before seasoning with salt.

3.   Remove squash from oven and with a fork using lengthwise strokes, separate the flesh. Add in the vegetable and lentil mixture and combine. Top with torn basil leaves, drizzle with any olive oil and lemon zest.

Asian Noodle Bowl

Servings: 2

Total Time: 15 minutes

Ingredients

- 4 ounces buckwheat soba noodles

- ½ cup broccoli florets, finely chopped

- ¼ head red cabbage, cored and thinly sliced

- ½ cup brussel sprouts, cored and thinly sliced

- 1 large carrot, shredded

- 1 scallion, sliced

- 2 tablespoons sesame seeds, toasted

- 1 tablespoon cilantro, chopped

Dressing

- ½ tablespoon ginger, minced

- 1 garlic clove, minced

- ½ tablespoon toasted sesame oil

- 2 teaspoons olive oil

- 2 tablespoons tamari

- 2 tablespoons coconut aminos

- ½ lime, juiced

- pinch of red pepper flakes

Directions

1.   Cook soba noodles according to package directions. Strain and rinse with cold water. Set aside.

2.   Make the Dressing by combining all Dressing ingredients and whisking well. Place vegetables and soba noodles in a large bowl and mix well to combine.

3.   Pour dressing over the noodles and vegetables. Sprinkle with sesame seeds, cilantro and serve.

Spicy Marinara Sauce & Pasta

Servings: 2

Total Time: 25 minutes

Ingredients

- 8 ounces spelt pasta
- 3 tablespoons olive oil
- 1 garlic clove, minced
- 1 shallot, diced
- 1 celery stalk plus greens, diced
- 1 carrot, diced
- 2 cups cherry tomatoes, diced
- ½ cup sun dried tomatoes, diced
- ½ small zucchini, diced
- ½ cup black olives, sliced
- 1 chili pepper, seeded and diced
- 1 teaspoon Himalayan salt
- 1 teaspoon black pepper, crushed
- 1 cup basil leaves, torn

Directions

1.   Cook spelt noodles according to package directions. Drain and set aside.

2.   Add oil to a medium skillet over medium heat and sauté the garlic and shallot for 3 minutes before adding the celery and carrot. Cook for an additional 8 minutes, stirring occasionally. Toss in cherry tomatoes, sun dried tomatoes and zucchini. Cook another 3 minutes. Stir in olives, chili pepper, salt and pepper.

3.   Toss pasta into the saucepan making sure to combine it thoroughly. Transfer to serving plate and top with basil leaves.

Lemon Baked Fish Over Green Salad

Servings: 2

Total Time: 30 minutes

Ingredients

- 8 ounces of wild salmon, cut into 2 fillets (skin on)
- ½ cup parsley, chopped
- ½ cup fresh basil, chopped
- 1 lemon, juiced
- 1 garlic clove, chopped
- 1 teaspoon cayenne pepper
- 1 tablespoon nutritional yeast
- 2 tablespoons olive oil
- 1 teaspoon sea salt
- 1 teaspoon black pepper, crushed
- ¼ cup pine nuts
- 4 lemon slices

Salad

- 3 cups kale, stems removed and sliced into thin ribbons
- 3 tablespoons olive oil

- 1 lemon, juiced

- 1 teaspoon Himalayan salt

- 1 cucumber, diced

- ¼ cup pepita seeds, toasted

- ½ avocado, diced

Directions

1.   Combine all ingredients except for the salmon and 4 lemon slices in a blender or food processor to form the greens mixture (add more olive oil if it is too thick).

2.   Place salmon on a parchment lined baking tray. Top each fillet with greens mixture and place 2 lemon slices on each piece. Bake salmon in a preheated 375°F/190°C oven for approximately 15-20 minutes or until fish flakes easily and is cooked all the way through.

3.   Place kale in a bowl and top with olive oil, lemon juice and salt. Massage the kale leaves until tender and set aside for 5 minutes before adding cucumber, pepitas and avocado.

4.   Serve fish alongside salad.

Cauliflower & Tahini Bowl

Servings: 2

Total Time: 30 minutes

Ingredients

- ½ head of cauliflower, chopped into small florets

- 1 tablespoon olive oil

- 1 teaspoon Himalayan salt

- 1 teaspoon black pepper, crushed

- 1 tablespoon coconut oil

- ½ cup cooked quinoa

- ¼ cup almonds, chopped

- ½ cup cilantro, chopped

- 1 tablespoon mint, chopped

- ½ cup watercress, chopped

Tahini Dressing

- 3 tablespoons tahini

- 1 tablespoon cashews, soaked overnight

- ¼ teaspoon cumin

- 1 garlic clove

- 1 lemon, juiced

- ¼ cup olive oil

- 1 teaspoon Himalayan salt

- 1 teaspoon black pepper, crushed

Directions

1.	Preheat oven to 425°F/220°C. Place cauliflower on parchment lined baking pan and drizzle with olive oil, salt and pepper. Roast for 15 minutes turning once halfway through.

2.	In a food processor, combine all the dressing ingredients and mix until creamy.

3.	Heat coconut oil in a skillet. Add quinoa, cooking 5 - 8 minutes or until toasted.

4.	In a large bowl add cauliflower, quinoa, almonds, cilantro, mint and watercress. Add in dressing and mix to combine.

Stuffed Peppers

Servings: 2

Total Time: 30 minutes

Ingredients

- 1 cup quinoa, cooked

- ½ cup green lentils, cooked

- 1 small red bell pepper, diced

- 1 small cucumber, diced

- ½ avocado, diced

- 2 tablespoons olive oil

- 1 teaspoon cumin

- 1 teaspoon chili powder

- ½ lime, juiced

- 1 tablespoon cilantro, chopped

- 1 teaspoon salt

- 1 teaspoon black pepper, crushed

- 2 small to medium bell peppers (assorted colors), tops cut off and seeds removed

Directions

1.   In a large bowl, combine the quinoa, lentil, diced bell pepper, cucumber and avocado.

2.   Whisk together the olive oil, cumin, chili, lime juice, cilantro, salt and pepper. Pour over quinoa lentil mixture and stir.

3.   Stuff each pepper with equal parts of the mixture.

Raw Beetroot Lasagna

Servings: 2

Total Time: 30 minutes

Ingredients

- ¾ cup cashews, soaked overnight and drained

- 1 teaspoon Himalayan salt

- 1 teaspoon pepper

- 1 teaspoon oregano

- 1 teaspoon dried basil

- ½ lemon, juiced

- 2 zucchinis, sliced thinly with a vegetable peeler

Beetroot Hummus

- 1 small beet, peeled and grated

- 2 cups chickpeas, cooked

- 2 tablespoons tahini

- 1 lemon, juiced

- 1 teaspoon cumin

- 1 teaspoon Himalayan salt

Directions

1.   In a food processor, combine cashews with salt, pepper, oregano, basil and lemon juice until smooth. Set aside and clean the food processor.

2.   Combine the beet, chickpeas, tahini, lemon juice, cumin and salt until creamy.

3.   In a deep baking dish create a layer of zucchini noodles. Top with Beet Hummus and then cashew mixture. Repeat until all ingredients are used.

4.   Chill 15 minutes before serving.

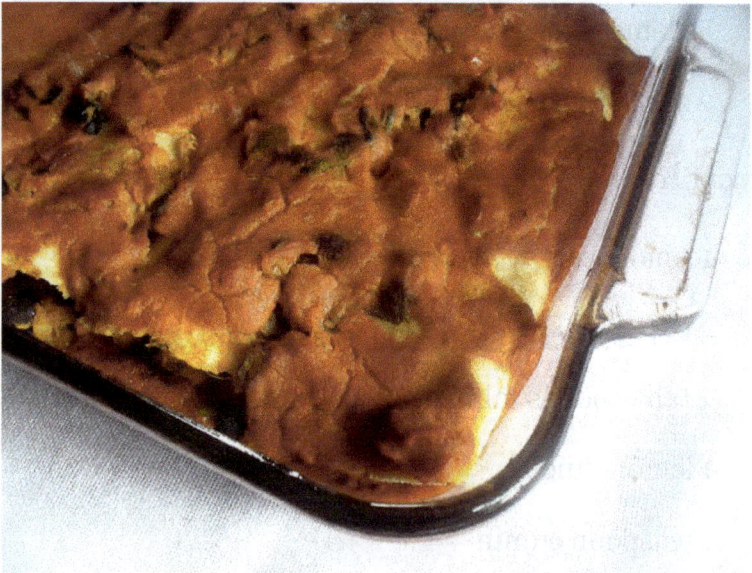

Baba Ganoush Pasta

Servings: 2

Total Time: 35 minutes

Ingredients

- 6 ounces spelt pasta
- 1 tablespoon olive oil
- 1 eggplant, cubed
- 1 zucchini, cubed
- ½ red bell pepper, cubed
- 1 medium-sized onion, chopped
- 1 garlic clove, minced
- 1 small chili pepper, seeded and chopped
- 1 cup vegetable stock
- 1/2 teaspoon Himalayan salt
- 1 pinch of cayenne pepper
- ¼ cup parsley, chopped

Directions

1. Cook pasta according to package directions. Set aside.

2.   Heat olive oil in a skillet and add eggplant, zucchini, pepper, onion, garlic and chili pepper. Cook for 5 - 8 minutes.

3.   Add vegetable stock and let cook another 3 - 5 minutes. Let cool before adding to blender and mixing until smooth.

4.   Return sauce back to skillet, season with salt and cayenne pepper. Toss in cooked pasta, sprinkle parsley and serve.

"Cheesy" Broccoli Bowl

Servings: 2

Total Time: 15 minutes

Ingredients

- 1 teaspoon olive oil

- 1 cup quinoa, cooked

- 4 cups broccoli florets, cooked

- 1 tablespoon lemon juice

- ¼ cup nutritional yeast

- ½ teaspoon Himalayan salt

- ½ teaspoon black pepper, crushed

Directions

1. In a skillet over medium heat add olive oil, cooked quinoa and broccoli. Cook for 5 minutes or until warmed.

2. Stir in lemon juice, nutritional yeast, salt and pepper.

3. Remove from heat and serve warm.

Lentil & Green Bean Pesto Salad

Servings: 2

Total Time: 20 minutes

Ingredients

- 2 cups green lentils, cooked

- 1 cup cherry tomatoes, halved

- 2 cups green beans, sliced into 1 inch pieces

- ¼ cup apple cider vinegar

- 2 tablespoons scallion (optional)

Pesto Sauce

- ¾ cup fresh basil leaves

- ½ cup spinach

- 2 tablespoons pine nuts

- 1 garlic clove, chopped

- ¼ cup olive oil

- 1 teaspoon Himalayan salt

Directions

1.   Combine Pesto ingredients in a food processor or blender until smooth and creamy.

2.   In a large bowl combine lentils, tomatoes, green beans, vinegar and scallions.

3.   Drizzle Pesto Sauce over the lentil mixture and toss well to coat before serving.

Vegetable Packed Minestrone

Servings: 2

Total Time: 20 minutes

Ingredients

- 1 tablespoon olive oil

- ½ cup of eggplant, cubed

- ½ cup of butternut squash, cubed

- ½ cup of zucchini, cubed

- ½ cup of carrot, diced

- 1 shallot

- 1 garlic clove, minced

- ½ cup kidney beans

- 1 cup of vegetable stock

- 1 cup of diced tomatoes

- 1 tablespoon oregano

- 2 teaspoons Himalayan salt

- 1 teaspoon black pepper

- 1 cup fresh basil

- 1 cup spinach

Directions

1.   In stock pot heat olive oil and add eggplant, squash, zucchini, carrot, shallot and garlic. Cook for 5 minutes, stirring occasionally.

2.   To the pot, add kidney beans, stock, diced tomatoes, oregano, salt and black pepper. Simmer another 10 minutes and season more to taste.

3.   Before serving, stir in basil and spinach.

Noodle Soup with Greens

Servings: 2

Total Time: 20 minutes

Ingredients

- 4 ounces soba noodles

- 2 cups water

- 1 ½ tablespoons coconut aminos

- 1 teaspoon ginger, grated

- ½ garlic clove, grated

- ¼ teaspoon Himalayan salt

- ½ cup shelled edamame beans

- ½ cup mushrooms, sliced

- ½ cup green peas

- ½ red bell pepper, sliced thin

- 1 ½ cups chopped baby bok choy - use both stems and greens

Directions

1. Cook soba noodles according to package directions.

2.   In a large stock pot, add water, aminos, ginger, garlic, salt, edamame, mushrooms, peas and bell pepper. Cook 15 minutes over medium low heat.

3.   Just before serving, stir in bok choy and cook 1 minute.

4.   Divide vegetables, broth and noodles evenly amongst two bowls.

Southwest Tofu Burger

Servings: 2

Total Time: 50 minutes

Ingredients

- 1 tablespoon olive oil

- ½ yellow onion, diced

- 1 cup green bell pepper, diced

- 1 carrot, diced

- 1 teaspoon Himalayan salt

- 1 teaspoon ground cumin

- ½ teaspoon ground cayenne pepper

- ½ teaspoon black pepper, crushed

- 4 ounces firm tofu, pressed between two heavy plates for at least 30 minutes

- 1 tablespoon nutritional yeast

- 1 tablespoon walnuts, finely crushed

- 1 tablespoon Dijon mustard

- 1 cup arugula

- 2 Bibb lettuce leaves

- 1 avocado, sliced

Directions

1. Heat olive oil in a medium skillet over medium-low heat. Add onion, bell pepper, carrot, salt, cumin, cayenne and black pepper. Cook for 5 - 8 minutes or until vegetables are soft.

2. Place vegetables in a bowl and let cool for 5 minutes. Discard liquid from the pressed tofu and grate tofu over the bowl. Add nutritional yeast, walnuts and Dijon mustard. Combine well until the mixture can be shaped into 2 burgers.

3. Preheat oven to 400°F/205°C. Place burgers on a baking tray lined with parchment paper. Bake for 30 minutes or until browned.

4. Allow to cool for 5 minutes then divide arugula between the lettuce leaves, top each with a burger and the sliced avocado.

Zucchini Rolls with Red Sauce

Servings: 2

Total Time: 50 minutes

Ingredients

- 1 tablespoon olive oil

- 1 yellow onion, finely chopped

- 3 Roma tomatoes, finely diced

- 1 red bell pepper, finely diced

- 1 teaspoon Himalayan salt

- 1 teaspoon dried oregano

- ¾ cup water

- 2 medium zucchinis, sliced into thin ribbons with a vegetable peeler

- 10 - 15 fresh basil leaves

Cashew Basil Filling

- 1 cup cashews, soaked overnight and drained

- 1 lemon, juiced

- 3 tablespoons water

- 1 tablespoon nutritional yeast

- ½ teaspoon Himalayan salt

- ¼ teaspoon black pepper, crushed

- ¼ teaspoon ground nutmeg

- 1 handful fresh basil, roughly chopped

Directions

1.　Heat oil in a medium skillet over medium heat. Add onion, tomato, bell pepper, salt and oregano to form the "red veggie mixture". Cook for 8 minutes or until vegetables are soft. Add water and let simmer for another 10 minutes. Transfer cooled vegetable mixture to food processor and blend until smooth.

2.　Place ingredients for the Cashew Basil Filling in the cleaned food processor and blend until smooth. This may take up to 10 minutes and you may need to add additional water to thin it out.

3.　Place zucchini ribbons on a platter in front of you and divide the Cashew Basil Filling amongst each ribbon. Roll up each zucchini ribbon tightly and place in a glass baking dish which has a light layer of the red veggie mixture spread on the bottom.

4.　Top each of the rolls with the remaining red veggie mixture and cook for 15 minutes in an oven that has been preheated to 375°F/190°C. Remove from oven and top each roll with fresh basil leaf.

Lentil, Walnut & Arugula Salad

Servings: 2

Total Time: 20 minutes

Ingredients

- 1 cup green lentils, cooked & drained
- 1 beet, roasted, peeled and diced
- ½ cup walnuts, toasted and chopped
- 2 cups arugula
- 2 teaspoons lemon zest

Mustard Dressing

- 1 tablespoon olive oil
- 1 tablespoon lemon juice
- 1 tablespoon Dijon mustard
- ¼ teaspoon salt
- ¼ teaspoon pepper

Directions

1.   In a large bowl combine lentils, beets, walnuts, arugula and lemon zest. Set aside

2.   Combine Dijon mustard and lemon juice in a small bowl. Slowly whisk in olive oil. Season with salt and pepper

3.   Pour Mustard Dressing over lentil salad and combine. Let sit at least 10 minutes before serving.

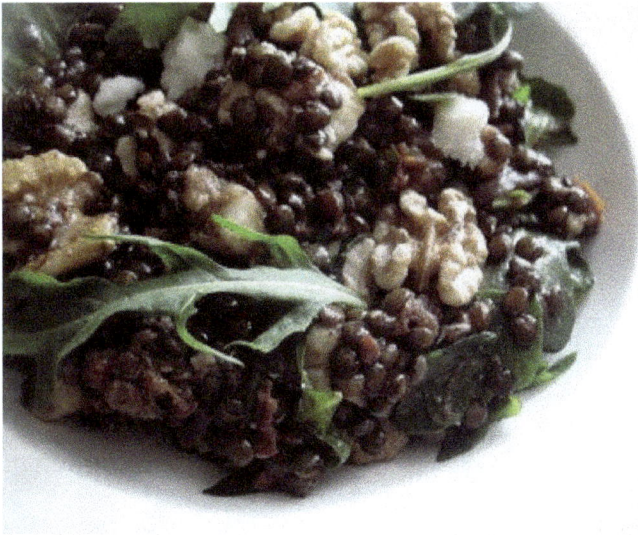

www.ingramcontent.com/pod-product-compliance
Lightning Source LLC
Chambersburg PA
CBHW050755030426
42336CB00012B/1822